Roberto Tsuneo Cervato Sato

Brachial plexus anesthesia for orthopedic surgery

Roberto Tsuneo Cervato Sato

Brachial plexus anesthesia for orthopedic surgery

Use of racemic bupivacaine (S50-R50) and 50% enantiomeric excess (S75-R25), technique with neurostimulation

ScienciaScripts

Imprint

Cover image: www.ingimage.com

This book is a translation from the original published under ISBN 978-613-9-67677-4.

Publisher:
Sciencia Scripts
is a trademark of
Dodo Books Indian Ocean Ltd. and OmniScriptum S.R.L publishing group

120 High Road, East Finchley, London, N2 9ED, United Kingdom
Str. Armeneasca 28/1, office 1, Chisinau MD-2012, Republic of Moldova, Europe
Printed at: see last page
ISBN: 978-620-8-17618-1

CONTENTS

INTRODUCTION

Localization of the brachial plexus can be done by direct contact of the needle with the nerve, when the patient reports paresthesia, despite the possible damage caused by direct contact with the nerve being approached. The use of a peripheral nerve stimulator, which uses an electric current that passes through the nerve and triggers contraction and movement of the muscle group innervated by the stimulated nerve, without the need for direct contact with the nerve, has been increasingly used. More recently, ultrasound has also been used to locate the nerves (CHAN, 2003; SALA-BLANCH 2004). The brachial plexus can still be located using anatomical references (IMBELLONI, 2005), the loss of air resistance technique (GEIER, 2004), X-rays and computed tomography (SALA-BLANCH, 2004), even fluoroscopy with image intensifier and contrast injection with local anaesthetic (NISHIYAMA, 1999). Magnetic resonance imaging has also contributed to the study and identification of the anatomical structures of the brachial plexus by adjusting established techniques (KLAASTAD, 2004; KLAASTAD, 2005).

There are many drugs available for anesthetizing the brachial plexus, and in addition to the multiple types of local anesthetics, each one has its own characteristics, and it is also possible to manipulate their isomeric composition, which results in the selection of different pharmacological characteristics for each isomeric portion, while maintaining the physicochemical characteristics (SIMONETTI, 1999; ZAPATA-SUDO, 2001; TRACHEZ, 2005; CHEDID, 2006).

For several decades, bupivacaine has been widely and successfully used in regional anesthesia for long-term procedures, providing excellent sensory blockade. However, some reports of unexpected accidents with the use of bupivacaine (ALBRIGHT, 1979; HEATH, 1982) have stimulated the search for safer alternatives with regard to cardiovascular complications, as well as central nervous system (CNS) toxicity (SIMONETTI, 1999).

Racemic bupivacaine is made up of an equimolar mixture of two enantiomers: R(+) and S(-) bupivacaine (VALE, 2000), containing 50% of each isomer, R(+) being the dextrorotatory form and S(-) the levorotatory form, i.e. if each enantiomer were isolated, the drug solution would deflect polarized light to the right and left, respectively (BURKE, et al. 2002). Starting from the purified isomers of the local anesthetic molecule, the enantiomeric ratio of a racemic compound can be manipulated. The aim is to help increase its efficacy and reduce its potential toxicity, thereby increasing the therapeutic index (FOSTER, 2000; SIMONETTI, 2000). The levomycin form is known to have lower cardiac toxicity (VANHOUTTE, 1991; MAZOIT, 1993; GRAF, 1997) and CNS toxicity (DENSON, 1990; DENSON, 1992), but lower potency (DENSON, 1992; MAZOIT, 1993; GRISTWOOD, 1994; COX, 1998; SIMONETTI, 1999; SIMONETTI, 2000; FOSTER, 2000; CHANG, 2000; D'AMBROSIO, 2001; CREWS, 2002; TANAKA, 2003).

MEE50% bupivacaine (S75-R25) at 0.5%, like the other formulations, has already been duly registered in the country and is on the market. The point is to evaluate its efficacy and the quality of the sensory and motor blockade for upper limb surgery, since its greater safety is widely reported in the national and international literature.

With regard to the safety of the drug, it can be said that it is not a new drug, but a controlled distribution of isomers, and that the extremes already tested, racemate (DELFINO, 1999b; IMBELLONI, 2002) and bupivacaine levogen (DELFINO, 1999a; DELFINO, 1999c; DELFINO, 2000; NAKAMURA, 2000; DELFINO, 2001a; DELFINO, 2001b), which ensured that the patient was not exposed to any additional risk; on the contrary, he benefited from this new isomeric combination, since the toxic portion for the cardiovascular system was reduced (VANHOUTTE, 1991; MAZOIT, 1993; GRAF, 1997; COX, 1998; SIMONETTI, 1999; CHANG, 2000; SIMONETTI, 2000; FOSTER, 2000; D'AMBROSIO, 2001; CREWS, 2002; TANAKA, 2003) and the nervous system (VANHOUTTE, 1991; MAZOIT, 1993; GRAF, 1997; COX, 1998; SIMONETTI, 1999; CHANG, 2000; SIMONETTI, 2000; FOSTER, 2000; D'AMBROSIO, 2001; CREWS, 2002; TANAKA, 2003). MEE50% bupivacaine (S75-R25) at 0.5% has been used in the anesthesia of children from 1 to 5 years old (IMBELLONI, 2002), ophthalmic anesthesia, with injection into the orbit until it spreads to the optic, oculomotor, abducens and trochlear nerves (SOARES, 2002), in anesthesia for cesarean sections, including with minimal fetal repercussions (DELFINO, 1999c; NAKAMURA, 2000), neuroaxis anesthesia with direct contact with the spinal cord (IMBELLONI, 2002) and epidural space (TANAKA, 2003), lower limb blocks with levobupivacaine (COX, 1998; CHANG, 2000; CREWS, 2002;

D'AMBROSIO, 2001) and finally in outpatient anesthesia (SOARES, 2002), all with proven safety and effectiveness.

From the point of view of cardiovascular and central nervous system toxicity, racemic bupivacaine is more toxic and can represent a serious complication (CHANG, 2001), with risk of death, if the drug is injected INADVERTEDLY into a blood vessel or into the central nervous system, specifically intrathecally in high doses compared to the usual doses for this site, since the intrathecal dose is much lower than the epidural dose or other peripheral segmental block, and can occur even with the precautionary measures recommended in the literature (SATO, 2000; SATO, 2001; SATO, 2003; SATO 2004).

OBJECTIVE

The aim of this study was to compare 0.5% MEE50% and 0.5% racemic bupivacaine in brachial plexus block for orthopaedic procedures on the upper limbs.

Brachial plexus block has been widely used in upper limb surgery with 0.5% racemic bupivacaine (S50-R50), which was then compared with 0.5% MEE50% bupivacaine (S75-R25) in terms of safety and efficacy.

In terms of complications, possible cardiovascular and neurological toxicity reactions were evaluated, as well as any other unexpected reactions.

Sensory and motor latency times were assessed up to the thirtieth minute, which was fundamentally the aim of the study.

Hemodynamic parameters such as heart rate and blood pressure were also compared between the groups.

ANATOMY OF THE BRACHIAL PLEXUS

The brachial plexus is made up of the ventral roots from C5 to T1, with a small contribution from the roots of C4 and T2 (figure 1).

The 5th and 6th cervical nerves join to form the superior trunk, which continues until it becomes the main component of the lateral cord. The ventral root of the 7th cervical nerve becomes the middle trunk and together with portions of the upper and lower trunk continues until it becomes the posterior cord. Finally, the ventral roots of the 8th cervical nerve and the 1st thoracic nerve form the inferior trunk which, together with portions of the middle trunk, becomes the median cord.

The brachial plexus crosses the scalene cleft near the surface between the anterior and middle scalene muscles. The formations or divisions in the individual cords described above occur under the clavicle and continue towards the axillary region, becoming individualized in each nerve as it continues towards the distal region (figure 2).

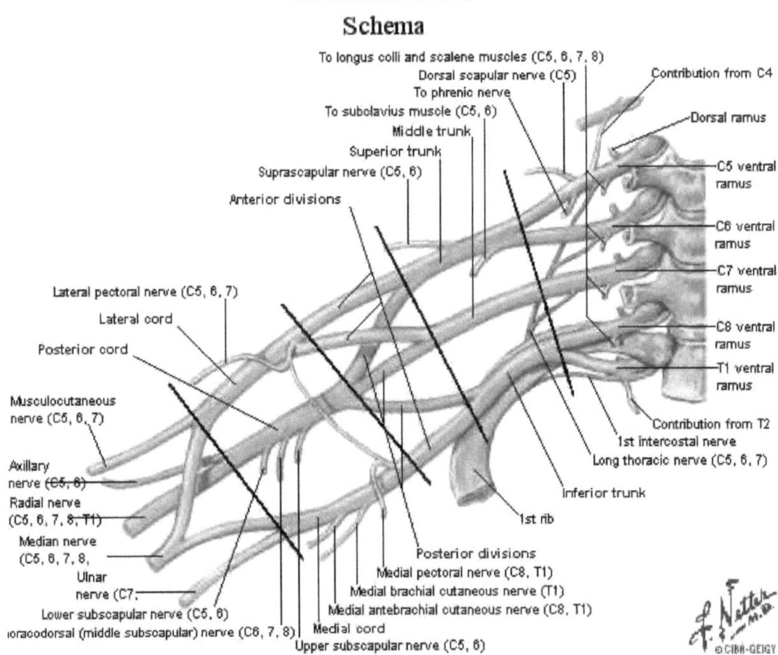

Figure 1 - Anatomy of the brachial plexus (NETTER, 1995), *by* Ciba-Geigy®.

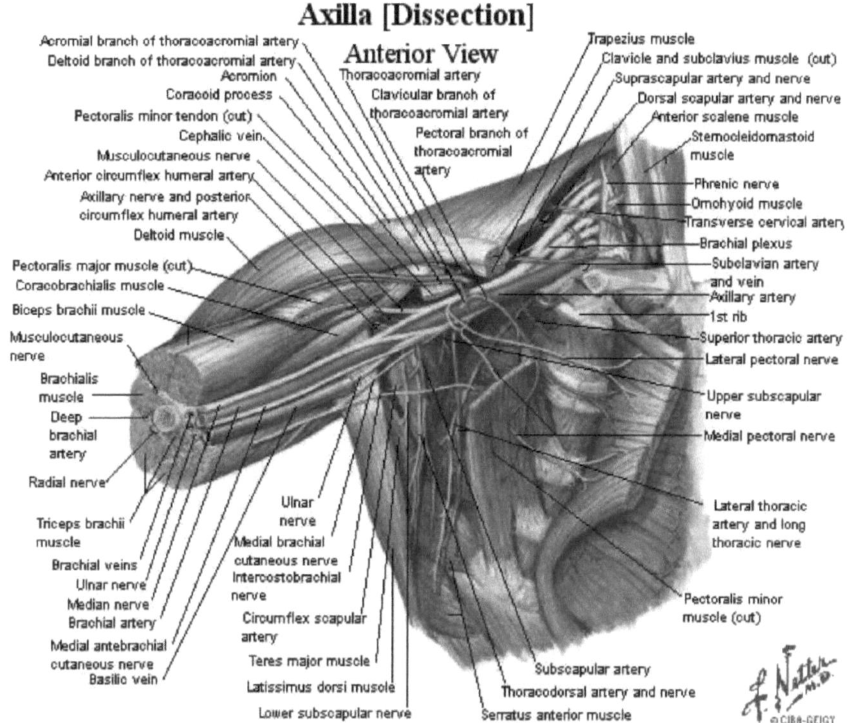

Figure 2 - Dissection of the brachial plexus in the axillary region (NETTER, 1995), by Ciba-Geigy.

The axillary artery together with the cords is wrapped in a common structure that runs under the clavicle in the direction of the axilla. This vascular and nerve sheath runs from the deep cervical fascia to the axillary fascia. Before reaching the axilla, the plexus divides into the following nerves:

. Musculocutaneous nerve, lateral cord.

. Median nerve, lateral and medial cord.

. Ulnar nerve, medial cord.

. Radial, axillary and humeral circumflex nerves of the posterior cord.

The multiple septation of this common sheath is attributed to the individual variation in the anesthetic response of the nerves, as it offers a barrier to the diffusion of the anesthetic to all compartments (THOMPSON, et al. 1983; PARTRIDGE, et al. 1987; NEAL, et al. 2002).

The motor innervation of the upper limb with the function of each muscle is listed in table I:

Table I - Innervation and function of the muscles of the upper limb

Peripheral nerve	Muscle	Function
Axillary	Deltoid	Arm abduction
Musculocutaneous	Biceps brachii Coracobrachial	Supine elbow flexion
Average	Flexor carpi radialis	Fist flexion and abduction
	Flexor digitorum brevis	Forearm pronation and proximal phalanx flexion
	Flexor digitorum profundus (I to III)	Flexion of the distal phalanges (I to III)
Radial	Triceps	Elbow extension
	Extensor carpi radialis	Wrist extension and abduction
	Finger extensors	Hand and finger extension Separating the fingers
Ulnar	Flexor carpi ulnaris	Wrist flexion and adduction
	Flexor digitorum profundus (IV to V)	Flexion of the distal phalanges (IVaV)

The sensory innervation of the upper limb and its cutaneous representation (figure 3a and b):

Cutaneous Innervation of Upper Limb

Anterior [Palmar] View

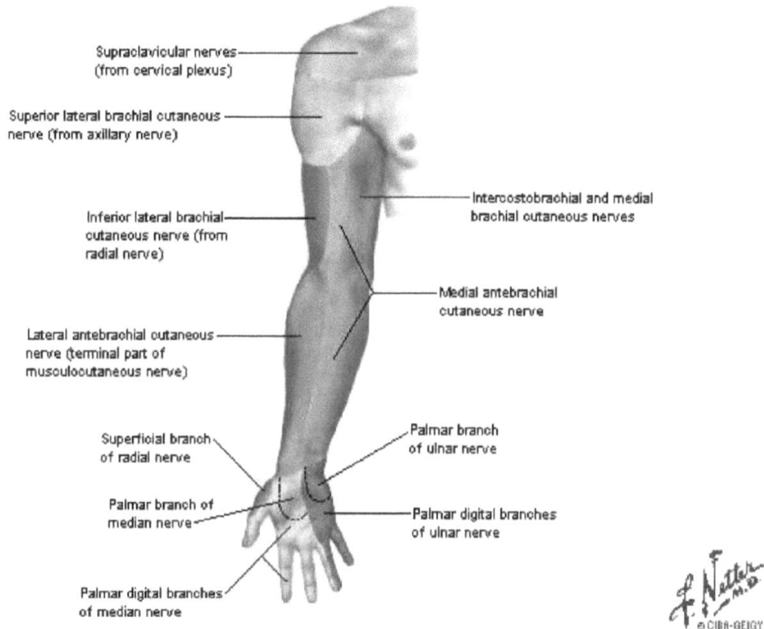

Figure - 3a: Sensory innervation of the upper limb, cutaneous projection.

Anterior view (NETTER, 1995), by Ciba-Geigy®.

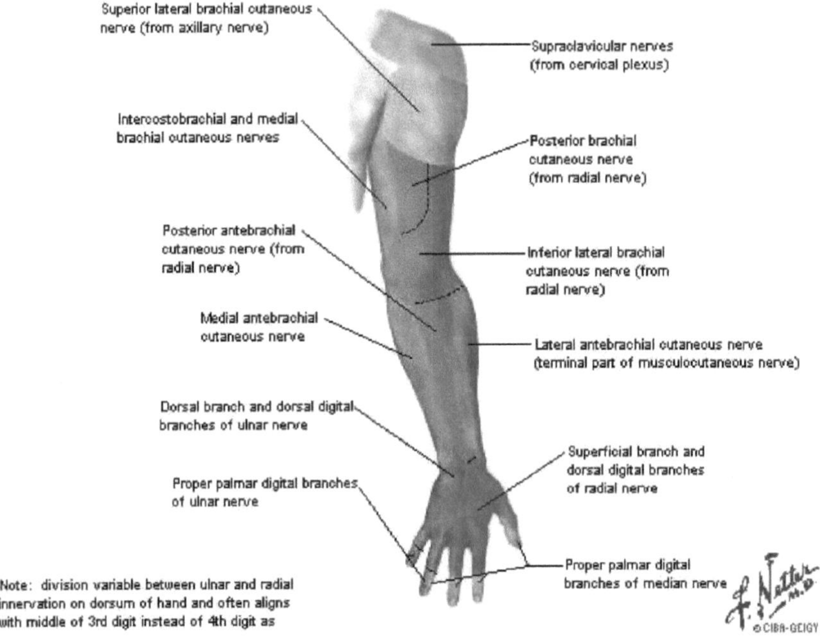

Figure - 3b: Sensory innervation of the upper limb, cutaneous projection.

Rear view (NETTER, 1995), by Ciba-Geigy®.

The motor innervation of the upper limb is illustrated in figure 4:

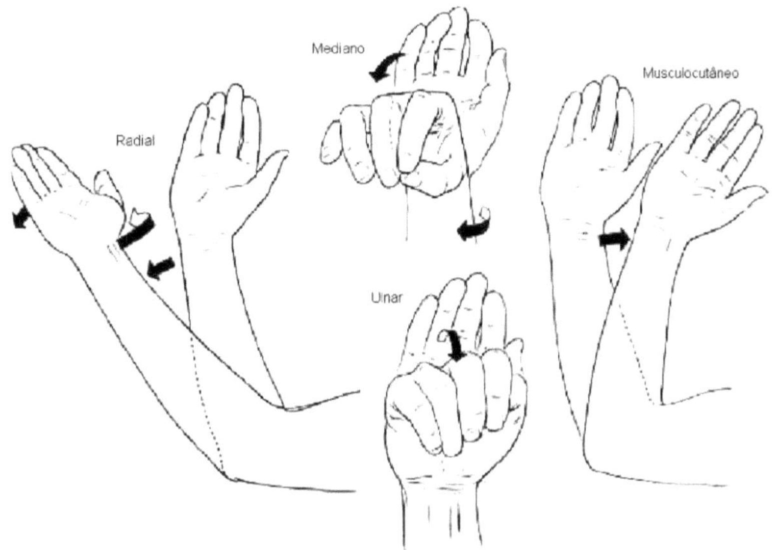

Figure 4 - Movements corresponding to the innervations of the upper limb (COUSINS, 2012).

CHIRALITY

The isomeric portions of a drug are unique molecular entities composed of the same molecular constituents with common structural characteristics. Stereoisomers are isomers of atoms, or groups of atoms, which differ by the structural arrangement of the ligands, they can be geometric or optical. Geometric isomers are stereoisomers without optically active centers and result from restricted rotation as a result of the presence, for example, of a carbon-carbon double bond (cis-2-butane, trans-2-butane). Geometric isomers are not mirror images of each other. For these compounds the terminology cis (meaning 'together' or 'same side') and trans (meaning 'opposite side') are used to describe spatial arrangements. Optical isomers are a subdivision of isomers that possess optical activity and have a chiral center.

The term 'chiral' comes from the Greek chiros, meaning 'hand', and describes a molecule that cannot be superimposed by its mirror image (figure 5). This is the definition of a molecule described as chiral (BURKE, et al. 2002).

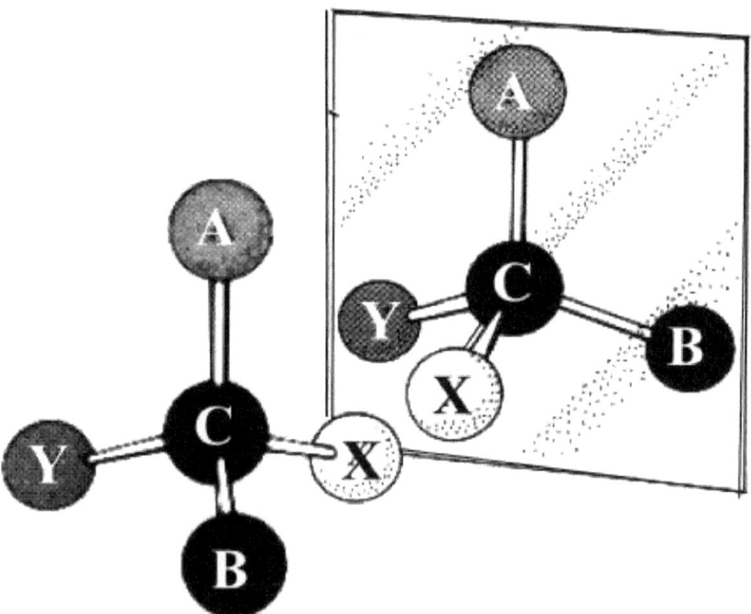

Figure 5 - Schematic representation of a molecule and its mirror shape (GRAF, 1998).

Optical isomerism establishes the existence of enantiomers (from the Greek *enantios* = opposite, *meros* = part) that share identical physical and chemical properties, but differ in terms of the plane of rotation of polarized light. They can also differ in their pharmacological action, having highly stereospecific interactions with the receptor, i.e. despite the same chemical constitution, one of the enantiomers has more affinity for a particular receptor.

When the stereoisomer, with its three-dimensional conformation, perfectly matches the receptor, it is called a 'eutomer', while a stereoisomer that only partially matches the receptor is called a 'distomer' (figure 6):

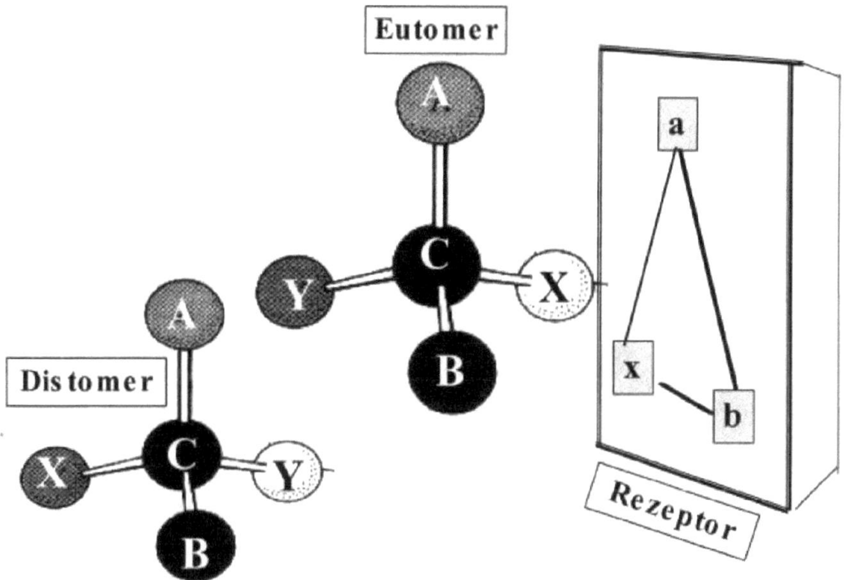

Figure 6 - Schematic representation of the combination between the eutomer and the receptor, and the impossibility of a complete combination of the distomer (GRAF, 1998).

Three bonds with the receptor, versus two bonds (figure 7):

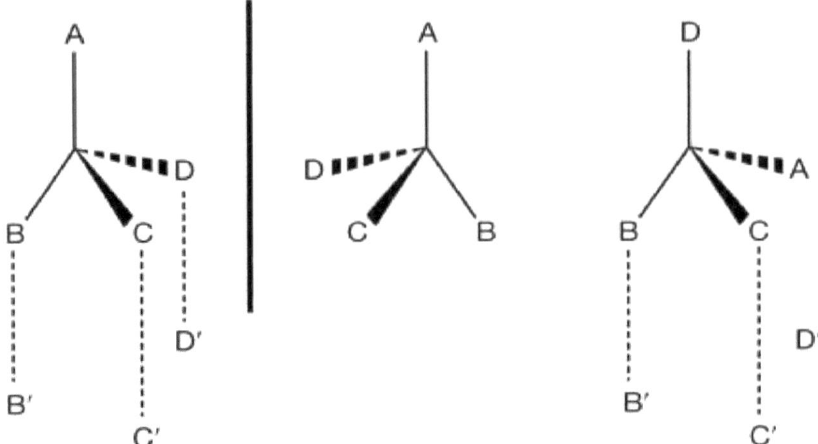

Figura 7 - Easson-Stedman model. The enantiomer on the left has three simultaneous bonds with the receptor, while the one on the right has only two. A, B, C and D represent ligands in the chiral compound and A', B', C' and D' are corresponding sites in the receptor (BURKE, et al. 2002).

Recently, Mesecar and Koshland (MESECAR, et al. 2000) proposed a new four-site interaction model. The three-site model described above assumes that the protein has a flat shape. Taking into account the protein's three-dimensional structure with an irregular surface, the three-site model may not be sufficient to allow or explain enantiomer interaction (figure 8).

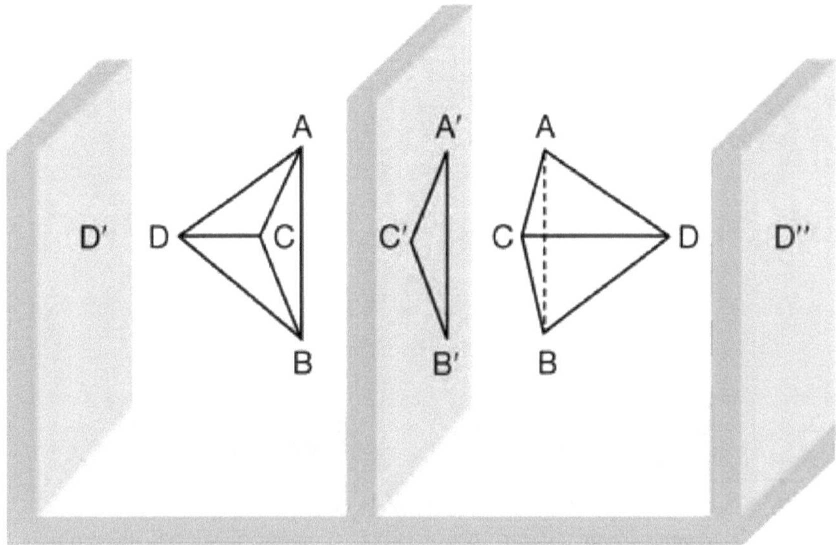

Figura 8 - Four-site model. This is a four-site model of protein stereoselectivity. Groups A, B and C of different isomers occupy the same site on the protein (A', B' and C'), while Group D, on the opposite side, interacts at different sites (D' and D'') (BURKE, et al. 2002).

A mixture of two enantiomers is called a 'racemate', or racemic mixture. The racemate is designated by the prefix (±) or rac-, or by the symbol RS or SR, and has no optical activity (BURKE, et al. 2002).

Relative description

The most common way of referring to a chiral molecule is still based on the rotation of the polarized light, (+) clockwise or (-) anti-clockwise (figure 9). Isomers that deflect the polarized light in a clockwise or anti-clockwise direction are called 'dextro-rotatory' and 'levo-rotatory' respectively.

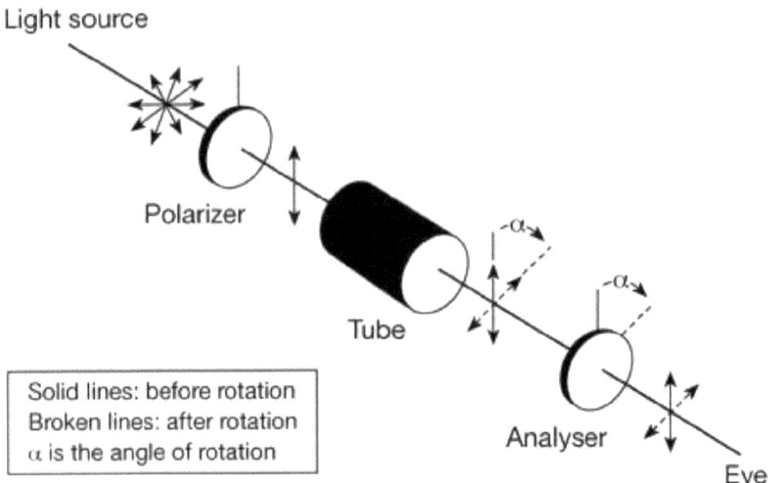

Figura 9 - Measurement of optical activity using a polarimeter (BURKE, et. al 2002).

Absolute description

This description is based on the molecular weight, according to the atomic number, of the radicals attached to the central chiral atom (figure 10). Consider the molecule C abcd, where a, b, c and d are groups located around the central C atom. If the sequence of ligands in terms of molecular weight, from largest to smallest, produces a clockwise progression, the arrangement is called 'R' from the Latin *rectus (right).* Similarly, if the progression is anticlockwise, it is called 'S' from the Latin *sinister (left).* Any chiral molecule can be classified in this way. If two or more ligands have the same molecular weight, the next atom in the chain is examined. Furthermore, a complete description of a chiral compound expresses the combination of terms from the absolute and relative description and the chemical name, for example, bupivacaine S(-).

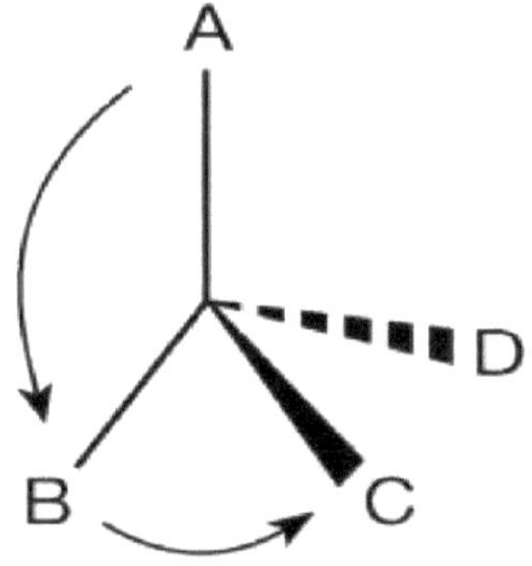

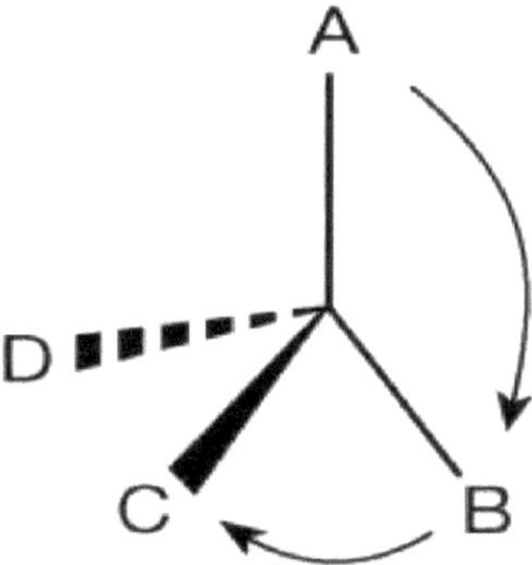

Figura 10 - Sequence rule. Bonds represented by solid lines are in the plane of the page, dotted lines project away, and wedged lines project towards the reader. Atomic weight is indicated as A>B>C>D, A representing the largest radical. The enantiomer in which the sequence is counterclockwise is designated 'S', and the enantiomer in which the sequence is clockwise, 'R' (BURKE, et. al 2002).

Definitions of enantiomers and their acronyms

- Racemic bupivacaine (RS, SR, rac-, ±):

- 50% of the bupivacaine isomer **in dextrographic** form
- 50% of the bupivacaine isomer in the **yeast** form

- Mixture with enantiomeric excess of bupivacaine (S75: R25) - MEE50%*:

- 75% of the bupivacaine isomer in the **yeast** form
- 25% of bupivacaine isomer **in dextrographic** form

*MEE50%: Based on the racemic mixture, there is a 50% excess of the levorotatory isomer.

- Bupivacaine levorate (S, -):

- 100% of the bupivacaine isomer in the **yeast** form

- Bupivacaine dextrograph (R, +):

- 100% of the bupivacaine isomer **in dextrographic** form

METHOD

Some aspects of the nerve stimulation method, in terms of the needles, the stimulator, the physiology of the sensory and motor nerve fibers and the anesthetic approach are described below.

Needles

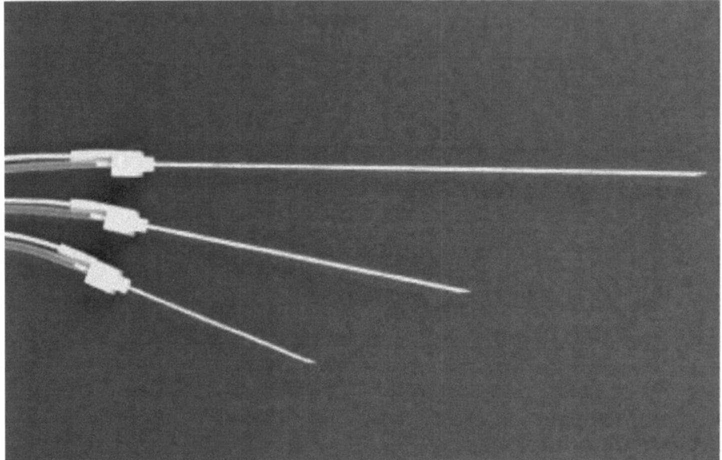

Figure 11 - Stimulation needles, B.Braun®.

The needles used are completely sheathed, electrically insulated, with the exception of a small area at the tip. This type of needle is called monopolar or unipolar. The electric current has a small outlet at the opening. Because of this, the electric field is directed and generates a high current density at the tip of the needle.

As soon as the needle approaches the nerve, the current required for depolarization drops. If the needle tip passes beyond the nerve, this value starts to rise again. This method makes it possible to locate the nerve exactly, while keeping the risk of direct nerve damage to a minimum.

Various opinions prevail regarding the role of the needle bevel and the risk of nerve damage. The use of needles with a short bevel (45°) in this work supposedly increases the level of safety, reducing the risk of nerve damage.

The procedure

- Testing the function of the nerve stimulator.

- Apply electrode and check for proper contact.
- Skin antisepsis.
- Placement of sterile drapes.
- Infiltration of the skin with anesthetic, taking care not to be so excessive as to reduce the effect of the nerve stimulator, with partial blockade.
- Connect the 20 ml syringe of local anesthetic to the 50 mm needle thread, flush with local anesthetic, connect the current wire and complete the circuit by connecting the stimulator's ground wire to the skin electrode.
- Set the nerve stimulator to a frequency of two Hz and a current of one mA.
- Puncture the skin and advance the stimulation needle into the subcutaneous tissue.
- Advance the needle towards the nerve until the muscle responds. While the response to the stimulus was being monitored, the current was reduced to 0.4 mA. At this stage it is important that the anesthesiologist and the assistant coordinate their activities. The assistant makes the adjustments while the anesthesiologist looks for a response to the stimulus by adjusting the position of the needle.
- If a visible contraction of the target muscle continued to occur at the proposed current, careful negative test aspiration was performed and the local anesthetic was injected.
- The stimulator current was set back to 1.0 mA and another contraction of the muscle group corresponding to another nerve was sought, the current was reduced and negative aspiration was repeated for a new injection of local anesthetic, until all the proposed nerves were reached.

Peripheral nerve stimulator

One of the advantages of the stimulator is that it doesn't depend on information from the patient to perform the block, and the patient can be sedated, unless it's a purely sensitive nerve. And the risk of nerve damage is minimal (figure 12).

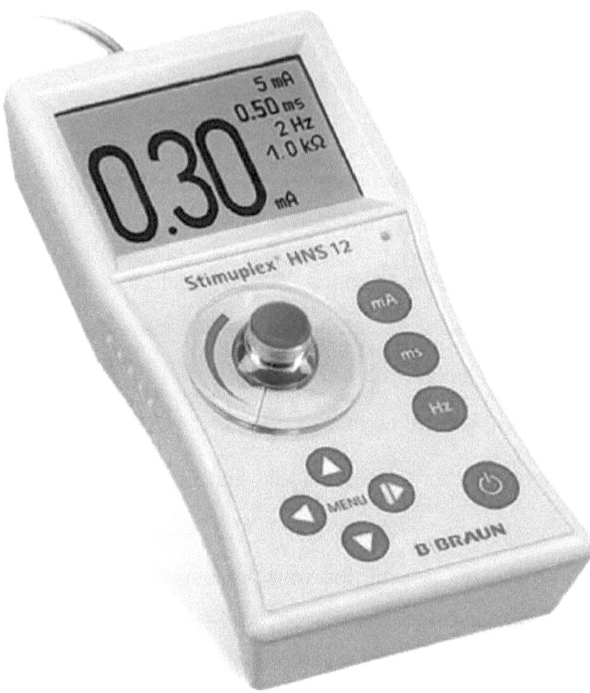

Figure 12 - Peripheral nerve stimulator used, Stimuplex HNS12®, Manufacturer BBraun®, Germany.

Neurophysiology and electrical nerve stimulation

The basic principle for understanding peripheral nerve stimulation is the electrophysiological properties of nerves and muscles.

Every living cell exhibits an internal voltage of around -90mV in relation to the external side of the membrane. This potential is called

'resting potential', and is maintained by an active balance of sodium and potassium ion concentrations between the two sides of the membrane (figures 13a, 13b and 14a and b).

Nerve and muscle cells have the ability to create short electrical impulses, called 'action potentials', in response to appropriate stimuli. A stimulus causes a depolarization of the membrane (decreases the membrane potential). Action potentials (nerve impulses) are of uniform amplitude, approximately 120mV (figures

13a and 13b).

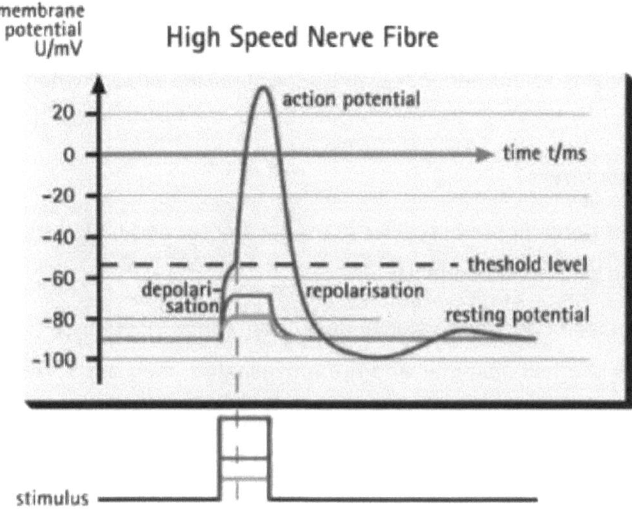

Figure 13a - Once the stimulus exceeds a certain intensity (resting potential), an action potential is generated and propagated along the nerve cell membrane. Especially along the nerve fiber that connects to other nerves or muscles.

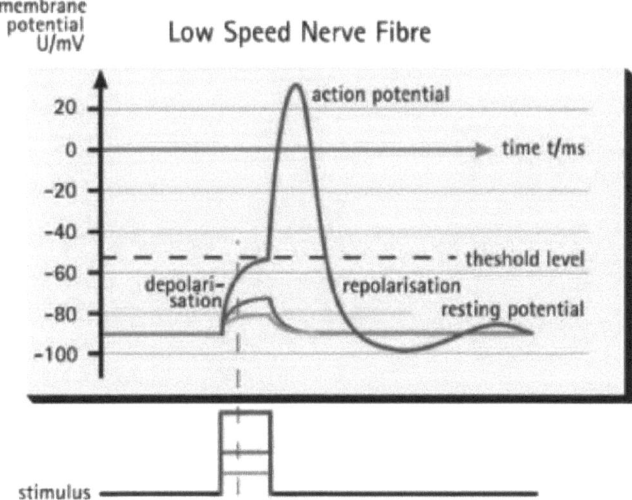

Figure 13b - Deflagration of the action potential in a low-speed nerve fiber.

Depending on the intensity and duration of the stimulus, a series of action potentials are generated while the amplitude of the stimulus is mainly represented by the frequency of the nerve impulses. In this way the information is decoded and transmitted to the CNS via the periphery. In the CNS the information is processed and via motor neurons returns to the periphery where the muscles are activated to move the body.

Sensory and motor nerve fibers

There are several types of nerve fibers that differ in their diameter and myelination, and have different impulse propagation speeds.

Nerve fibers with low impulse conduction velocity (less than 1 $m.s^{-1}$), such as pain fibers (visceral pain) have a small diameter and are amyelinated, they are 'C' type fibers. Fast conducting fibers (greater than 120 $m.s^{-1}$) are the motor fibers of the limb muscles, for example, and have a larger diameter and are myelinated, they are 'A - delta' type fibers (DE ANDRES, 2001) (figure 14a and b).

Nerve fibre (Axon) with insulation (myelin sheath)
e.g. motor fibre

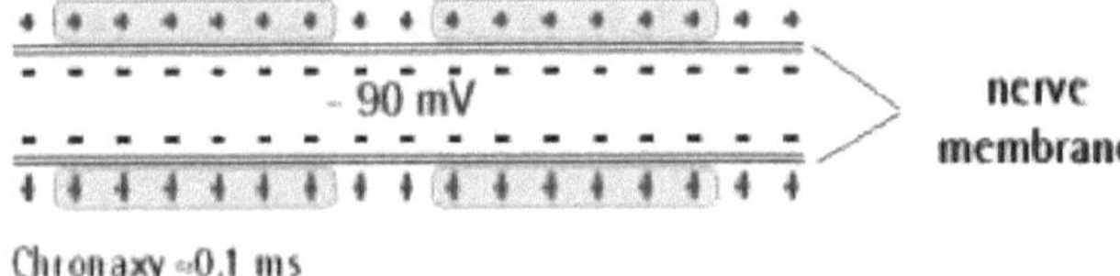

Nerve fibre (Axon) without insulation,
e.g. pain fibre

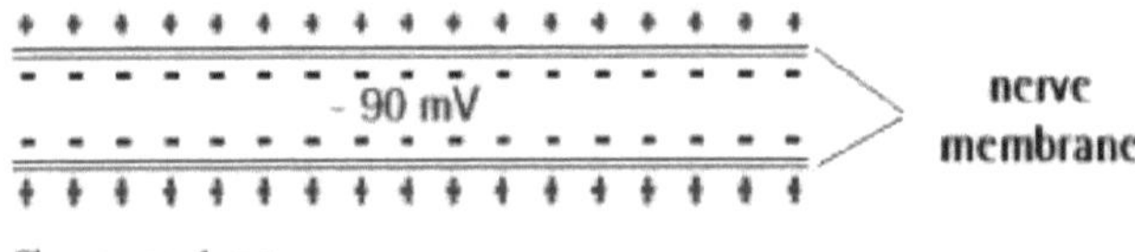

Figures 14a and b - Timing of motor (myelinated) and sensory (amyelinated) nerve fibers, respectively.

In addition to the differences in the speed of nerve impulse propagation, nerve fibers also differ in their excitability to external electrical stimulation, with myelinated fibers requiring a greater charge to propagate compared to myelinated nerve fibers. This means that a longer stimulation time is needed to reach the resting threshold and trigger the action potential (figures 13a and 13b).

Rheobase and Chronaxis

Rheobase is defined as the smallest stimulus amplitude (intensity) capable of triggering a stable action potential (DE ANDRES, 2001; HADZIC, 2003).

Chronaxia is defined as the shortest stimulus duration capable of promoting an action potential with an amplitude of twice the rheobase (DE ANDRES, 2001; HADZIC, 2003). An electrical stimulus with the duration of chronaxia is very effective in promoting an action potential. If the stimulus duration is too short, the stimulus may not trigger an action potential even at a higher amplitude; pain fibers are not excited by a 0.1ms stimulus (figure 14a and b).

The nerve approach with the stimulation needle

The amount of current, or charge, received by the nerve membrane depends primarily on the distance between the needle tip and the nerve. This means that the reaction of the muscle, innervated by the target nerve, when the needle is approaching increases and the current can be decreased again to the resting threshold.

The situation is illustrated in figure 15a and 15 b, step by step the current is decreased while approaching the nerve until the desired current (usually between 0.2 and 0.5 mA with 0.1 ms stimulation duration) is reached. The tip of the needle is then close enough to the nerve to inject the local anesthetic, but still at a safe distance so as not to injure the nerve by direct contact or even intraneural injection.

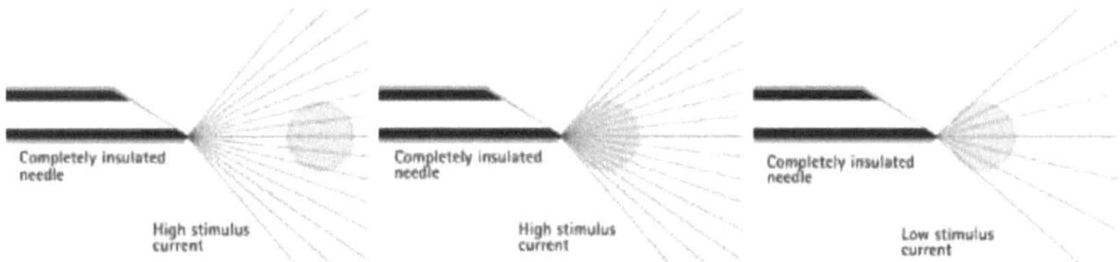

Figures 15a, b and c - The amount of current reaching the nerve increases as the needle approaches, reaching the resting threshold when the intensity of the stimulus decreases.

Methodology

After approval by the Research Ethics Committee of the Pontifical Catholic University of Paranà PUCPR, 40 consecutive patients took part in the randomized, prospective, double-blind study (the person who prepared the local anaesthetic solution was someone else, so they didn't know what the solution was or which group the patient belonged to), aged between 18 and 90 years, with ASA class I and II physical status, undergoing orthopaedic surgery of the upper limbs. Patients with peripheral neuropathy, hypersensitivity reactions to bupivacaine, sepsis, anatomical deformities in the cervical region, morbid obesity and lung disease were excluded.

The patients were divided into two equal groups according to the local anesthetic administered: Group L - patients who received MEE50% bupivacaine (S75-R25) at 0.5%; and Group R - patients who received racemic bupivacaine at 0.5%, both with adrenaline 1:200,000. They received a pre-anesthetic visit the night before surgery, during which their physical condition was assessed and permission to take part in the study was requested. The following morning, in the operating room, after local anesthesia with 2ml of 1% lidocaine, the patients underwent venoclysis with a 20G or 18G catheter in the upper limb contralateral to the surgical site. Monitoring consisted of routine cardioscopy in the DII shunt, non-invasive blood pressure measurement and pulse oximetry. All patients received oxygen under face mask 8 l.min^{-1} , midazolam 2 mg and fentanyl 50mcg intravenously.

The double puncture technique, interscalene and axillary, was used. The interscalene puncture (at the level of the cricoid cartilage) was performed with the patient in the supine position and with the head turned to the side contralateral to the puncture and the arm positioned parallel to the trunk, preceded by antisepsis and placement of surgical drapes for infiltration of the skin and subcutaneous cellular tissue with 1 ml of the solution to be used. The injection site was identified using a peripheral nerve stimulator (Stimuplex®) with an A50 needle, set at 1 mA initially with a frequency of 2 Hz, reduced to 0.4 mA while maintaining muscle stimulation of the corresponding nerve fraction. Half of the proposed volume was injected.

The axillary puncture was performed immediately afterwards with the patient in the same position, except for the arm which was perpendicular to the trunk, exposing the axillary cavity. The puncture site was based on palpation of the brachial artery as proximal as possible and the same procedures were followed as for the interscalene block with injection of the second half of the proposed volume, always with negative aspiration for blood or cerebrospinal fluid, the latter in the interscalene puncture.

The neurostimulation affected 4 nerve portions, corresponding to the radial nerve, elbow extension; the musculocutaneous nerve, elbow flexion; the median nerve, wrist flexion; and the ulnar nerve, thumb adduction, if not in the interscalene puncture, then in the axillary puncture (PERRIS 2003). During the surgical procedure, additional fractional doses of midazolam were administered intravenously for sedation after the 30-minute initial assessment. The total volume of anesthetic used was set at 0.6 $ml.kg^{-1}$ ($3mg.kg^{-1}$), limited to 40 ml, half of which was used at each of the two puncture sites.

Moment zero (0) was defined as immediately after the end of the punctures; moments 5, 10, 15, 20, 25 and 30 corresponded to the time in minutes after the axillary puncture. At these times, heart rate, blood pressure, sensory and motor blockade were assessed. The duration of the double punctures was three minutes on average.

The protocol for assessing motor blockade was muscle contractions of the areas innervated by muscle groups that corresponded to movements similar to neurostimulation (JANZEN, et al. 2001; BORGEAT, et al. 2001). Patients were asked to extend the elbow to assess radial nerve block; flex the elbow, musculocutaneous nerve; flex the wrist, median nerve; and adduct the thumb, ulnar nerve (figure 4). The degree of motor blockade was defined as zero (0) when there was no blockade at all, one (1) when there was partial blockade and two (2) when the blockade was total.

The protocol for assessing the sensory block was painful stimulation with a 14x8 needle in the areas of cutaneous innervation corresponding to each nerve (JANZEN, et al. 2001; BORGEAT, et *al.* 2001). The areas were stimulated, with questioning and observation of the patients' faces, in the dorsal region between the 1st and 2nd metacarpal, to assess radial nerve block; lateral region of the forearm, musculocutaneous nerve; ventral region of the 2nd metacarpal, median nerve; medial region of the forearm, medial cutaneous nerve of the forearm and hypothenar region, ulnar nerve (figure 3). The degree of sensory blockade was defined as zero (0) when sensitivity was normal, one (1) when there was analgesia and two (2) when there was surgical anesthesia. When the patient reported sensitivity level 1, it was compared with the contralateral side to check whether or not sensitivity levels 0 and 2 were different.

All the complications and complications that occurred during the follow-up period were recorded, as defined below (TANAKA, et al. 2003): Mediate - muscle tremors, tinnitus, drowsiness, psychomotor agitation, cardiac dysrhythmia, convulsion, arterial hypotension greater than 30% of the initial systemic pressure, heart rate less than 50 bpm. Late (24 hours after surgery), pain at the injection site, inflammation at the injection site, areas of anesthesia and motor deficit. The parametric Student's t test and the non-parametric Mann-Whitney U test were used to verify the objectives of the study, when appropriate.

We opted for the double block, which is routine in this anesthesiology teaching and training center, due to the profile of trauma patient care, as there is a need to reduce the failure rate as much as possible, which is higher when using simple puncture, in order to minimize the risk of bronchoaspiration of gastric contents when the block fails and the need for deep sedation or conversion to general anesthesia.

The toxicity limit of 0.5% racemic bupivacaine solution or MEE50% 0.5% bupivacaine (S75-R25) has been set at 3 $mg.kg^{-1}$ (BARDSLEY, et al. 1998) or 0.6 $ml.kg^{-1}$, both with adrenaline 1:200,000 as the dose to be used. The presence of adrenaline at this concentration, 5 $mcg.ml^{-1}$, reduces systemic absorption by around a third (STOELTING, 1997), promoting vasoconstriction at the injected site, interfering with the speed of absorption of the drug, causing it to remain there longer, in contact with the nerve roots (GOUVEIA, et al., 2000).

There are no studies in the literature that look at the enantiomeric mixture under the same conditions, which leads us to consider other studies involving the pure levorotatory enantiomer in situations similar to this one.

RESULTS

A total of 40 patients were enrolled and none were withdrawn from the study. There were no statistically significant differences between the two groups in terms of age, weight, height, gender and physical condition (Table II).

Table II - Demographic Data

		Group R (n=20)	**GroupL** (n=20)
Age (years)	Median	39,5	43,5
	Minimum and maximum	18 - 69	18 - 90
Weight (kg)	Mean ± SD	73,40 ± 6,46	71,50 ± 7,72
	Minimum and maximum	66 - 90	53 - 85
Height (m)	Mean ± SD	1,70 ± 0,09	1,69 ± 0,08
	Minimum and maximum	1,54 - 1,89	1,60 - 1,81
Sex	Male	13	13
	Female	7	7
Physical state	ASA I	15	13
	ASA II	5	7

There was no significant difference between the groups ($p < 0.05$).

The distribution of surgeries by group was similar (table III).

Table III - Distribution of surgeries by site of intervention.

	Group R	**Group L**
Mao	6	5
Fist	7	7
Forearm Elbow	6 0	6 1
Arm	0	1

The total volume of local anesthetic used, as well as the duration of the surgery, did not differ between the groups (Table VI).

Table VI - Volume used and duration of surgery.

		Group R (n=20)	Group L (n=20)
Volume (ml)	Mean ± SD	37,9 ± 3,34	38,5 ± 3,09
	Minimum and maximum	30 - 40	30 - 40
Duration (minutes)	Median surgery	85	90
	Minimum and maximum	60 - 240	60 - 150

There was no significant difference between the groups (p< 0.05).

Systolic blood pressure was higher in group R, with a statistically significant difference, and remained the same as the surgery progressed. Diastolic blood pressure evolved without statistical difference. There were no cases of bradycardia or hypotension (graphs 1, 2 and 3).

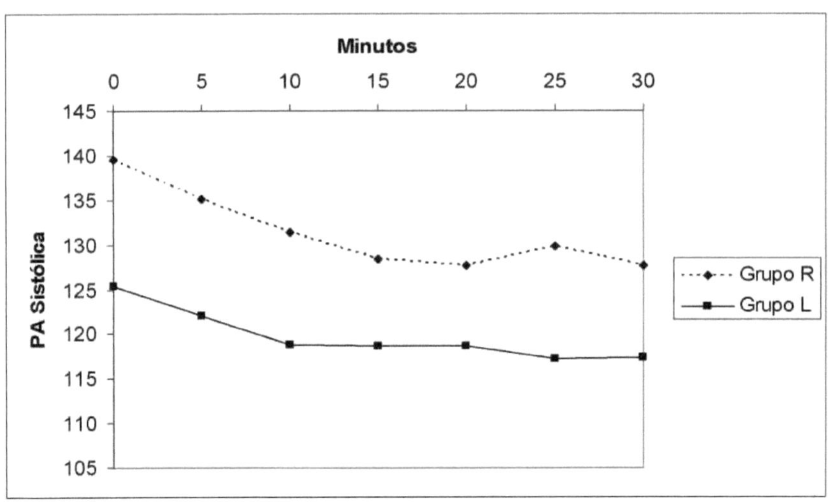

Graph 1 - Systemic blood pressure (mmHg) at different times in the study groups.

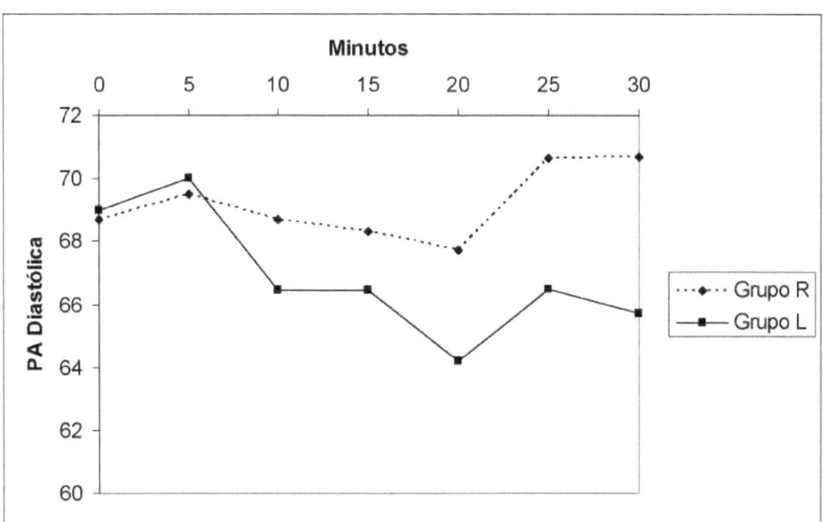

Graph 2 - Diastolic blood pressure (mmHg) at different times in the study groups.

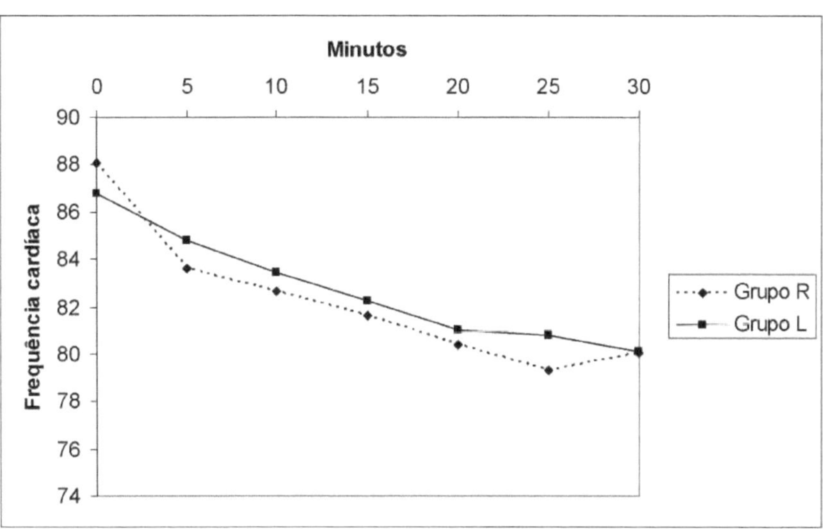

Graph 3 - Average heart rate (bpm) at the different times in the groups studied.

There were no cases of total anesthesia failure, defined as the absence of a total motor or sensory block of zero (0) at time 30 in the corresponding area of innervation. All cases had at least one (1) sensory or motor block at time 5 in the corresponding area of innervation. The sensory and motor latency time in each corresponding innervation area did not result in a statistically significant difference, with the exception of the motor latency corresponding to the ulnar nerve area (table V and graphs 4 and 5).

Table V - Average Sensitive and Total Motor Lock Time (min).

		Group R (n=20)	**Group L** (n=20)
Sensory block			
	N. Musculocutaneous	7,75 (7'45")	7 (7'00")
	N. Radial	7,5 (7'30")	7 (7'00")
	N. Median	9 (9'00")	8,25 (8'15")
	N. Ulnar	8,5 (8'30")	8 (8'00")
	N. Lateral cutaneous forearm.	6,75 (6'45")	7,5 (7'30")
Motor lock			
	N. Radial	6 (6'00")	8,25 (8'15")
	N. Musculocutaneous	8,25 (8'15")	9 (9'00")
	N. Median	13 (13'00")	14,25 (14'15")
	N. Ulnar*	**10,75 (10'45")**	**14,25 (14'15")**

- There was a significant difference between the groups (p< 0.05).

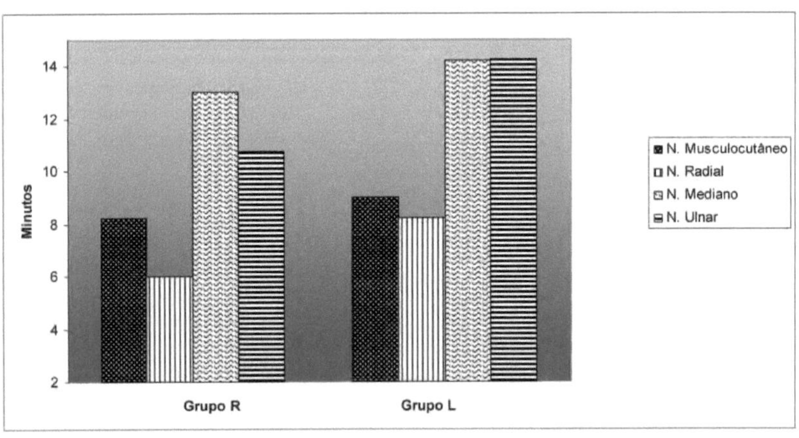

Graph 4 - Average motor latency time for each nerve in both groups.

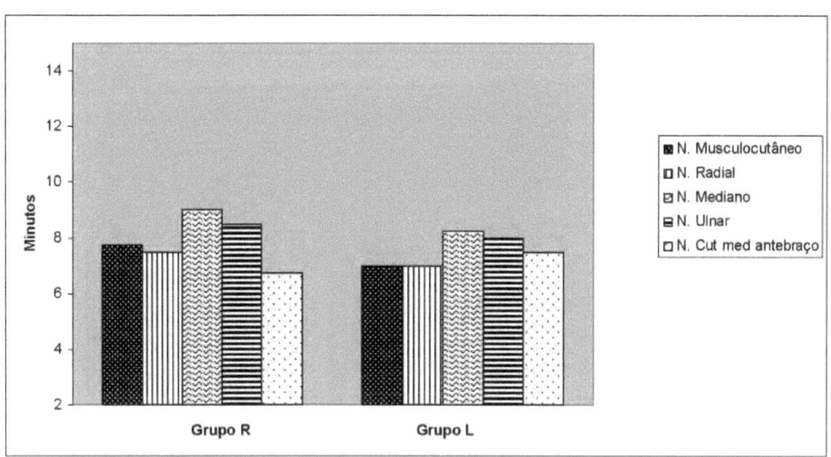

Graph 5 - Average Sensory Latency Time for each Nerve in both Groups.

When comparing the time course of total sensory blockade in the two groups, there was no statistically significant difference (graphs 6 and 7).

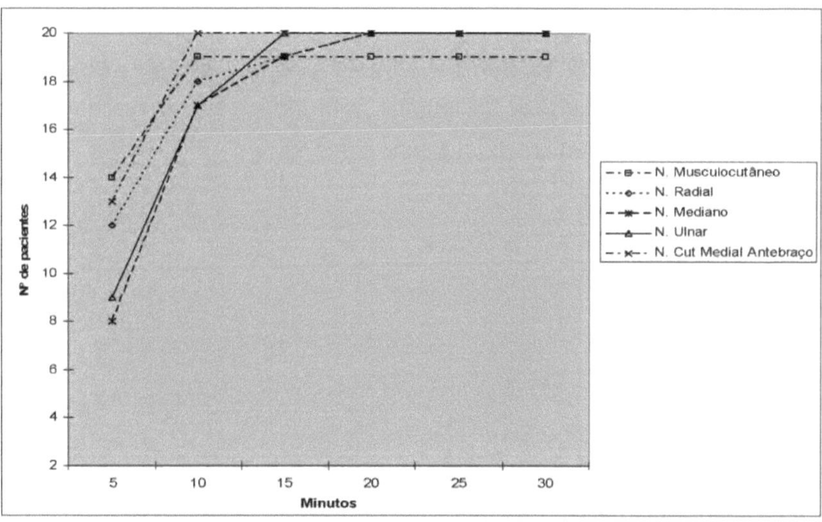

Graph 6 - Evolution of the Total Sensory Blockade of each Nerve Studied in Group R.

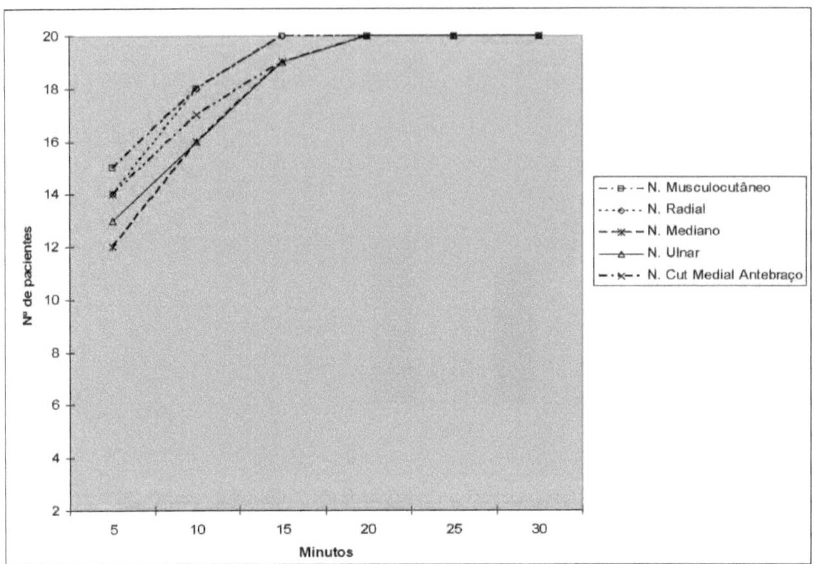

Graph 7 - Evolution of the Total Sensory Blockade of each Nerve Studied in Group L.

When comparing the temporal evolution of total motor blockade in the two groups, there was no statistically significant difference, with the exception of ulnar nerve blockade, which was greater in group L (graphs 8 and 9).

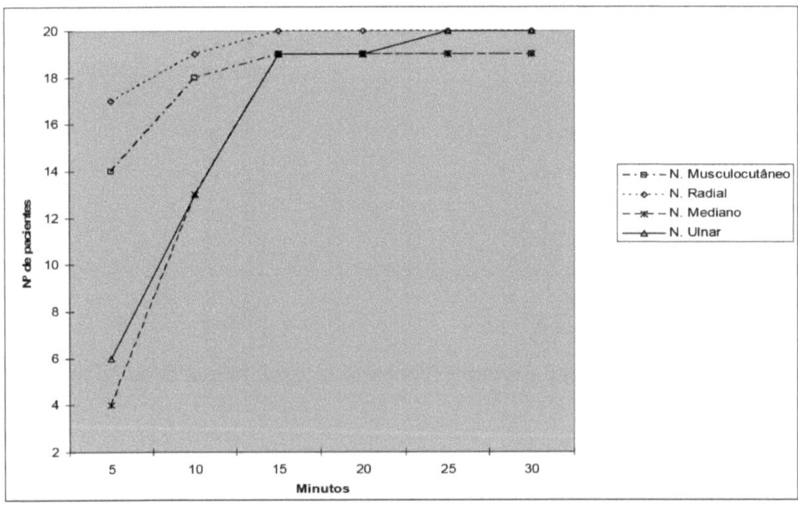

Graph 8 - Evolution of the Total Motor Blockade of each Nerve Studied in Group R.

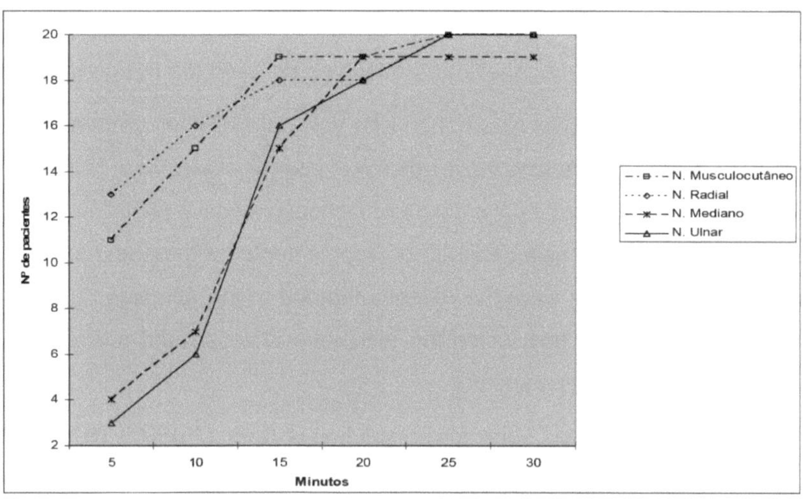

Graph 9 - Evolution of the Total Motor Blockade of each Nerve Studied in Group L.

Regarding the efficacy of the two drugs, we found that in the thirtieth minute the rate of total sensory and motor anesthesia was satisfactory. If we consider that in the **motor** evaluation, the radial, musculocutaneous, median and ulnar nerves were evaluated in the thirtieth minute in the twenty patients, we conclude that there were 80 evaluations. As for the **sensory** evaluation, we added the medial cutaneous nerve of the forearm, resulting in 100 evaluations at the same time (Table VI).

Table VI - Total sensory and motor efficiency in the thirtieth minute in both groups.

Groups	Type evaluation	ofSuccess (%)	30th minute evaluations (#)	Faults	
				Nerves	Location
R	Sensitive	99	100	1	N. Musculocutaneous
	Engine	97,50	80	2	N. Musculocutaneous and N. Ulnar
L	Sensitive	100	100	0	-
	Engine	98,75	80	1	N. Median

The success may have been even greater, since the complete blockade may have occurred after the thirtieth minute, which was not evaluated.

DISCUSSION

In this study, demographic homogeneity was observed between the two groups.

The profile of care at the hospital where the study was carried out is trauma, which means that it is necessary to reduce the incidence of poor blocks or block failures as much as possible. This is to reduce the risk of bronchoaspiration of gastric contents, which can occur when anesthesia needs to be supplemented with deeper sedation or general anesthesia. These were the reasons that led to the adoption of double puncture as the service's routine, since the technique is associated with a lower incidence of failures than single puncture.

The safety limit of 0.5% racemic bupivacaine solution or 0.5% MEE50% (S75-R25) with 1:200,000 epinephrine was set at 3 mg.Kg^{-1} (BARDSLEY, et al. 1998) or 0.6 ml.kg^{-1} . The presence of epinephrine at this concentration, 5 µg.ml^{-1} , reduces systemic absorption by a third (STOELTING, 1997), as a result of vasoconstriction at the injection site, with a slower rate of absorption of the drug, causing it to remain there longer, in contact with the nerve roots (GOUVEIA & LABRUNIE, 2000).

In the literature consulted, no study was found that included MEE50% for brachial plexus blockade, and this study is unprecedented in the literature indexed in Medline and Scielo. However, it is possible to compare it with other studies that have used the pure levorotatory enantiomer in situations similar to this one. In a study comparing racemic and 0.5% levorotatory bupivacaine in the brachial plexus, no difference was found in the success rate (COX, et al., 1998).

In this study, the two groups behaved similarly, with no statistically significant difference in total sensory and total motor latency times. Only the mean total motor latency for the ulnar nerve was longer in group L, with a statistically significant difference. However, this mean difference of 3.5 minutes (3'30") is not clinically relevant.

The latency of 12.5 minutes (12'30") for the sensory block in the axillary block with 0.5% levobupivacaine from a reference surveyed (CREWS, 2002) corroborates the present study, although in this one the double block and MEE50% at 0.5% (S75-R25) with epinephrine 1:200,000 were used, leaving a latency of 7.55 minutes (7'33").

In another study (D'AMBROSIO 2001), in the brachial plexus, the time to start surgery was similar in the two groups, racemic bupivacaine and 0.5% levocaine, corroborating the results of the present study.

Recent studies suggest that intravascular injection and systemic toxicity are more common in peripheral regional anesthesia techniques (HORLOCKER 2002). The search for a long-acting local anesthetic, with less potential for toxicity and effective motor and sensory blockade, even when compared to anesthetics that are already well-established, is therefore necessary, as the potentially fatal reactions to incidents with racemic bupivacaine are well known (ALBRIGHT, 1979; CHANG, 2001). Incidents with levobupivacaine have also been described (CREWS 2003), but with less toxicity (CHANG, 2000; KOPACZ, 1999; HUANG, 1998; SALOMAKI, 2005; KHAN, 2003; PIROTTA, 2002).

In the evaluation of hemodynamic parameters, there was no statistically significant difference in heart rate and diastolic blood pressure at the different times studied. However, there was a statistically significant difference in systemic blood pressure, which was higher in group R. It could be assumed that this difference is due to an intrinsic property of the drug in the racemic formulation, since the groups were demographically homogeneous, but further research is needed to prove this assumption.

Graf (GRAF, et al. 1997) showed that there is stereoselectivity between the bupivacaine enantiomers in terms of atrioventricular conduction time, with bupivacaine R(+) being more depressant, to the point of producing Mobitz II-type second-degree atrioventricular block in 75% of the hearts isolated for the study, while none occurred in the bupivacaine S(-) group, with only Mobitz I-type block in 8% of the hearts studied.

Chedid (CHEDID, et al. 2006) and colleagues have studied the effects of bupivacaine and its enantiomers at cellular level. They demonstrated the stereoselectivity of bupivacaine S(-) in increasing the intracellular calcium concentration of isolated cardiac cells by activating ryanodine receptors (RYR2) in the sarcoplasm more efficiently than bupivacaine R(+), which leads to less cardiac fiber depression.

Zapata-Sudo (ZAPATA-SUDO, et al. 2001) also demonstrated that there is stereoselectivity for the bupivacaine enantiomers, at a concentration of 10 μM, and found an increase in the PR interval and QRS duration of 80% and 370%, respectively, with bupivacaine R(+), and 25% and 200% for bupivacaine S(-). He attributed this difference to direct blockade of sodium channels and indirect blockade of potassium channels.

Similarly to the present study, Trachez (TRACHEZ, et al. 2005) studied the potency and toxicity of the mixture of enantiomers in the proportion of seventy-five percent in the form of bupivacaine S(-) and twenty-five percent in the form of bupivacaine R(+), 75S(-): 25R(+), the pure enantiomers, R(+) and S(-) and the racemate. The results found (Table VII) show that the 75S:25R mixture is safer than the others in terms of cardiac muscle recovery and lethal dose, as well as being effective in terms of motor blockade. The results corroborate this study in terms of effectiveness, since cardiac muscle recovery and lethal dose were not tested, but there was no sign of toxicity.

Table VII - Potency and toxicity of bupivacaine (TRACHEZ, et al. 2005).

75S :

	RS (±)	**25R**	**R(+)**	**S(-)**
RS-related motor block (±)	1,0	1,0	0,31	0,40
Lethal dose (2 mg.kg^{-1} .min)$^{-1}$	18	16	39	34
Cardiac muscle recovery (%)	43	75	38	69

Cases have been described of successful resuscitation from inadvertent intravenous injections of bupivacaine S(-), with no lethal hemodynamic repercussions or sequelae (KOPACZ, 1999; SALOMAKI, 2005). The same applies to signs of CNS intoxication, which are apparently milder and self-limiting (KHAN, 2003; PIROTTA, 2002).

CONCLUSION

Chirality

The possibility of manipulating enantiomers allows for the selection of desired drug characteristics, always seeking greater effectiveness with minimal toxicity. The mixture with an enantiomeric excess of bupivacaine (S75:R25) used in this study seems to point in this direction. The characteristics of effectiveness were maintained with no apparent cases of systemic toxicity.

Use of the peripheral nerve stimulator

The certainty of locating the peripheral nerve close enough to ensure the presence of local anesthetic involving the nerve is a premise for properly assessing the effectiveness of the anesthetic solution. At the same time, the integrity of the peripheral nerve is safeguarded, and there is no need for the needle to directly touch this structure, which can cause nerve trauma with nerve damage, which can be permanent.

This study

In this study, adequate motor and sensory blockade for surgery was observed in both groups, with no side effects or signs of toxicity, suggesting that the solutions are suitable for brachial plexus anesthesia for orthopedic surgery.

The lower toxicity of MEE50% bupivacaine (S75-R25) represents a safer alternative to racemic bupivacaine.

In a nutshell

- The two drugs behaved similarly:

- Sensory and motor latency time (efficiency):

• The exception was the ulnar nerve motor latency of 14'15" versus 10'45", a difference of 3'30", which was greater in the MEE50% group.

• Statistically significant, but clinically of little relevance.

- Hemodynamic parameters:

- The exception was systemic BP, which was higher in the racemic group.

MEE50% of 0.5% bupivacaine with 1:200,000 adrenaline is an effective and safe option for use in upper limb anesthesia, as well as having fewer hemodynamic repercussions.

REFERENCES

ALBRIGHT, G.A. Cardiac arrest following regional anesthesia with etidocaine or bupivacaine. **Anesthesiology**; 51: 285-287, 1979.

BARDSLEY, H.; GRISTWOOD, R.; BAKER, H.; WATSON, N.; NIMMO, W. A comparison of the cardiovascular effects of levobupivacaine and racemic bupivacaine following intravenous administration to healthy volunteers. **British Journal of Clinical Pharmacology**; 46: 245-9, 1998.

BORGEAT, A.; EKATODRAMIS, G.; DUMONT, C. An evaluation of the infraclavicular block via a modified approach of the Raj technique. **Anesth Analg**; Aug; 93(2): 436-41, 2001.

BURKE, D.; HENDERSON, D. J. Chirality: a blueprint for the future. **Br. J. Anaesth.** 88: 563-576, 2002.

CHAN, V. W. S.; PERLAS, A.; RAWSON, R. R. N.; ODUKOYA, O. - Ultrasound-Guided Supraclavicular Brachial Plexus Block. **Anesth Analg**. 97(5):1514-1517, 2003.

CHANG, D.H.; LADD, L.A.; WILSON, K.A. Tolerability of Large-Dose Intravenous Levobupivacaine in Sheep. **Anesth Analg**; 91:671-9, 2000.

CHEDID, N. G. B.; SUDO, R. T.; AGUIAR, M. I. S.; TRACHEZ, M. M.; MASUDA, M. O.; ZAPATA-SUDO, G. - Regulation of Intracellular Calcium by Bupivacaine Isomers in Cardiac Myocytes from Wistar Rats. **Anesth Analg.** 102(3):792-798, 2006.

COUSINS, M. J. Cousins and Bridenbaugh's Neural Blockade in Clinical

Anesthesia and Pain Medicine, 4ª Ed. Lippincott Williams & Wilkins, 2012.

COX, C.R.; CHECKETTS, M.R.; MACKENZIE, N. Comparison of S(-)- bupivacaine with racemic (RS)-bupivacaine in supraclavicular Brachial Plexus Block. **Br J Anaesth**; 80: 594-598, 1998.

CREWS, J.C.; ROTHMAN, T.E. Seizure After Levobupivacaine for Interscalene Brachial Plexus Block. Case Report. **Anesth Analg**; 96:1188-90, 2003.

CREWS, J.C.; WELLER, R.S.; MOSS, J.; JAMES, R.L. Levobupivacaine for axillary brachial plexus block: a pharmacokinetic and clinical comparison in patients with normal renal function or renal disease. **Anesth Analg**; 95(1):219-23, 2002.

D'AMBROSIO, A.; DE NEGRI, P.; DAMATO, A.; CAVALLUZZO, A.; BORGHI, B. S (-) bupivacaine (levobupivacaine) in peripheral blocks: preliminary results . **Minerva Anestesiol**; 67 (9 Suppl 1):37-43, 2001.

DELFINO, J.; VALE, N. B.; MAGALHAES FILHO, E. Comparison between Racemic Bupivacaine and 0.5% Levocaine. Study in Epidural Anesthesia for Varicose Vein Surgery. **Rev Bras Anestesiol**; 49: 1: 4 - 8, 1999a.

DELFINO, J.; PONTES, S.; GONDIM, D.; VALE, N. B. Comparative Study between 0.5% Bupivacaine and 0.5% Isobaric Ropivacaine in Subarachnoid Anesthesia for Orthopedic Surgery. **Rev Bras Anestesiol**; 49: 3: 160 - 164, 1999b.

DELFINO, J.; VALE, N. B.; MAGALHAES FILHO, E. Ropivacaine and Levobupivacaine at 0.45% Associated with Opioids in Epidural Anesthesia for Cesarean Section: Comparative Study. **Rev Bras Anestesiol**; 49: 4: 244 - 248, 1999c.

DELFINO, J.; VALE N. B. Bupivacaine Levogira at 0.5% Pure versus Enantiomeric Mixture of Bupivacaine (S75-R25) at 0.5% in Epidural Anesthesia for Varicose Vein Surgery. **Rev Bras Anestesiol**; 51: 6: 474 - 482, 2001a.

DELFINO, J.; VALE, N. B. Subarachnoid Anesthesia with 0.5% Isobaric Ropivacaine or Levobupivacaine in Lower Limb Surgeries. **Rev Bras Anestesiol**; 51: 2: 91 - 97, 2001b.

DENSON, D.; BEHBEHANI, M.; GREGG, R. Enantiomer specific effects of an intravenously administered arrhythmogenic dose of bupivacaine on neurons of the nucleus tractus solitarius and the cardiovascular system in the anesthetized rat. **Reg Anesth**; 17: 331-6, 1992.

DENSON, D. D.; BEHBEHANI, M. M.; GREGG, R. V. Effects of an intravenously administered arrhythmogenic dose of bupivacaine at the nucleus tractus solitarius in the conscious rat. **Reg Anesth**; 15: 76-80, 1990.

DENSON, D. D.; BEHBEHANI, M. M.; GREGG, R.V. Enantiomer-specific effects of an intravenously administered arrhythmogenic dose of bupivacaine on neurons of the nucleus tractus solitarius and the cardiovascular system in the anesthetized rat.

Reg Anesth; 17: 311-16, 1992.

FOSTER, R. H.; MARKHAM, A. Levobupivacaine: a review of its pharmacology and use as a local anaesthetic. Review. **Drugs**; Mar; 59(3):551-79, 2000.

GEIER, K.O. - The Loss of Resistance Technique: A New Paradigm in Interscalene Continuous Brachial Blockade? **Rev Bras Anestesiol**. v.54. (Supl 33), 2004.

GOUVEIA, M.A.; LABRUNIE, G. Factores que Influenciam o Bloque Peridural, in: Vale N, Delfino J - **Anestesia Peridural: Atualizaçao e Perspectiva**; Sâo Paulo, Editora Atheneu; 117-126, 2000.

GRAF, B. M.; MARTIN, E. - Stereoisomers in anesthesia. Theoretical basis and clinical relevance. **Der Anaesthesist**. 47:172-183, 1998.

GRAF, B. M.; MARTIN, E.; BOSNJAK, Z, J.; et al. Stereospecific effect of bupivacaine isomers on atrioventricular conduction in the isolated perfused guinea pig heart. **Anesthesiology**; 86: 410-19, 1997.

NETTER, F. H. **Interactive Atlas of Human Anatomy**. Editors Dalley, A.

F.; Myers, A. F. Ciba Medical Education & Publications, 1995.

GRISTWOOD, R.; BARDSLEY, H.; BAKER, H.; DICKENS, J. Reduced cardiotoxicity of levobupivacaine compared with racemic bupivacaine (Marcaine): new clinical evidence. **Exp Opin Invest Drugs**; 3: 1209-12, 1994.

HADZIC, A. ; VLOKA, J.; HADZIC, N; THYS, D.; SANTOS, A. Nerve Stimulators Used for Peripheral Nerve Blocks Vary in Their Electrical Characteristics **.Anesthesiology**, V 98, 4, 2003.

DE ANDRES J., SALA-BLANCH, X. Peripheral Nerve Stimulation in the Practice of Brachial plexus Anesthesia: A Review. **Reg Anesth and Pain Med** Vol. 26, No. 5 2001; pp478-483.

HEATH, M. Deaths after intravenous regional anesthesia. **BMJ**; 285: 913-4, 1982.

HORLOCKER, T.T.; WEDEL, D.J. Local Anesthetic Toxicity-Does Product Labeling Reflect Actual Risk? **Reg Anesth and Pain Med**; 27, No: 562-567, 2002.

HUANG, Y.F.; PRYOR, M.E.; MATHER, L.E.; VEERING B.T. Cardiovascular and central nervous system effects of intravenous bupivacaine and levobupivacaine in sheep. **Anesth Analg**; 86: 797-804, 1998.

IMBELLONI, L.E.; BEATO, L.; CORDEIRO, J.A.- Comparison of the Transarterial and Multiple Nerve Stimulation Techniques for Axillary Brachial Plexus Block Using Lidocaine with Epinephrine. **Rev Bras Anestesiol**, 55(1):40-49, 2005.

IMBELLONI, L.E.; VIEIRA, E.M.; BEATO, L.; SPERNI, F. Spinal Anesthesia with the Enantiomeric Mixture of Bupivacaine at 0.5% Isobaric (S75- R25) in Children Aged 1 to 5 Years for Outpatient Surgery. **Rev Bras Anestesiol**; 52: 3: 286 -293, 2002.

JANZEN, P.R.; VIPOND, A.J.; BUSH, D.J.; HOPKINS, P.M. A comparison of 1% prilocaine with 0.5% ropivacaine for outpatient-based surgery under axillary brachial plexus block. **Anesth Analg**. Jul; 93(1): 187-91, 2001.

KLAASTAD, O.; SMITH H. J.; SMEDBY, O.; ET AL. - A novel infraclavicular brachial plexus block: the lateral and sagittal technique, developed by magnetic resonance imaging studies. **Anesth Analg**;98:252-6, 2004.

KLAASTAD, O.; SMEDBY, O.; KJELSTRUP, T.; SMITH, H. - The Vertical Infraclavicular Brachial Plexus Block: A Simulation Study Using Magnetic Resonance Imaging. **Anesth Analg**;101(1):273-278, 2005.

KOPACZ, D.J.; ALLEN, H.W. Accidental intravenous levobupivacaine. **Anesth Analg** 89:1027-9, 1999.

MAZOIT, J.; BOICO, O.; SAMII, K. Myocardial uptake of bupivacaine. II. Pharmacokinetics and pharmacodynamics of bupivacaine enantiomers in isolated perfused rabbit heart. **Anesth Analg**; 77: 477-82, 1993.

MCLEOD, G. A.; BURKE, D. Levobupivacaine. **Anaesthesia**; April; Vol 56(4): pp 331-341, 2001.

MESECAR, A.D.; KOSHLAND, D. E. A new model for protein stereospecificity. **Nature; 403**: 614-5, 2000.

NAKAMURA, G.; CASTIGLIA, Y. M. M.; NASCIMENTO JÙNIOR, P.; RUGOLLO, L. M. S. S. Bupivacaine, Ropivacaine and Levobupivacaine in Labor Analgesia and Anesthesia. Maternal and Fetal Repercussions. **Rev Bras Anestesiol**; 50: 2: 105 - 111, 2000.

NEAL, J.M.; HEBL, J. R.; GERANCHER, J. C.; HOGAN, Q. H. Brachial plexus anesthesia: Essentials of our current understanding. **Reg Anesth & Pain Medicine**;27, 4, 402-428, 2002.

NISHIYAMA, M.; NAGANUMA, K.; AMAKI, Y. - A New Approach for Brachial Plexus Block Under Fluoroscopic Guidance. **Anesth Analg;** 88(1):91-97, January 1999

PARTRIDGE, B. L.; BENIRSCHKE, K.. Functional anatomy of the brachial plexus sheath: implications for anesthesia. **Anesthesiology**.;66:743-747, 1987.

PERRIS, T. M.; WATT, J. M. - The road to success: A review of 1000 axillary brachial plexus blocks. **Anaesthesia;** 58(12):1220-1224, 2003

PIROTTA, D.; SPRIGGE, J. Convulsions following axillary brachial plexus blockade with levobupivacaine. Case Report. **Anaesthesia**, 57, pg 1187-1189, 2002.

SALA-BLANCH, X.; DE ANDRES, J. - Image-guided techniques for peripheral nerve blocks. **Current Opinion in Anaesthesiology**. 17(5):409-415, 2004.

SALOMAKI, T.E.; LAURILA, P. A.; VILLE, J. - Successful Resuscitation after Cardiovascular Collapse following Accidental Intravenous Infusion of Levobupivacaine during General Anesthesia. **Anesthesiology**; 103:1095-6, 2005.

SATO, R. T. C. - Accidental intravascular injection of ropivacaine in epidural block. Case Report. **Rev Bras Anestesiol**; 51. p.168 - 168 (Supl), 2001.

SATO, R. T. C. - Accidental intravascular injection of ropivacaine in epidural block. Case report. **Rev Bras Anestesiol**; 53. (Supl), 2003.

SATO, R. T. C. - Total spinal anesthesia after interscalene brachial plexus block. Case Report. **Rev Bras Anestesiol**; 50: 3: 246 - 247, 2000.

SATO, R. T. C., OTTOBONI, L. S. - Total Spinal Anesthesia After Epidural Block During Inhalational General Anesthesia. Case Report. **Rev Bras Anestesiol**; 54. (Supl), 2004.

SIMONETTI, M. P. B. - Spinal Local Anesthetics, in: Vale N, Delfino J - **Anestesia Peridural: Atualizaçao e Perspectiva**, Sâo Paulo, Editora Atheneu; 81-92, 2000.

SIMONETTI, M. P. B.; BATISTA, R. A.; FERREIRA, F. M. C. - Stereoisomery: the interface of industrial drug technology and therapeutic rationalization. **Rev Bras**

Anestesiol; 48: 390-399, 1999.

SOARES, L. F.; HELAYEL, P. E.; CONCEIÇÂO, D. B.; OLIVEIRA FILHO, G. R. Peribulbar Block with the Association of the Enantiomeric Mixture of Bupivacaine (S75-R25) at 0.5% and Lidocaine at 2%: Effects of the Addition of Hyaluronidase. **Rev Bras Anestesiol**; 52: 4: 420 - 425, 2002.

STOELTING, R.K. **Pràtica Anestésica**, 1ª Ed. Porto Alegre, Editora Artes Médicas Sul: 109, 1997.

TANAKA, P.P.; SOUZA, R.O.; SALVALLAGIO, M.F.O. Comparative Study between 0.5% Bupivacaine and 0.5% Enantiomeric Bupivacaine Mixture (S75-R25) in Epidural Anesthesia in Patients Undergoing Lower Limb Orthopedic Surgery. **Rev Bras Anestesiol**; 53: 3: 331 - 337, 2003.

THOMPSON, G. E.; RORIE, D. K. Functional anatomy of the brachial plexus sheaths. **Anesthesiology**.;59:117-122, 1983.

TRACHEZ, M. M.; ZAPATA-SUDO, G.; MOREIRA, O. R.; CHEDID, N. G. B.; RUSSO, V. F. T.; RUSSO, E. M. S.; SUDO, R. T. - Motor nerve blockade potency and toxicity of non-racemic bupivacaine in rats. **Acta Anaesthesiol Scand**. 49(1):66-71, 2005

VALE, N.; DELFINO, J. - Pharmacology of Local Anesthetics, in: Vale N, Delfino J - **Anestesia Peridural: Atualizaçao e Perspectiva**, Sâo Paulo, Editora Atheneu; 41-64, 2000.

VANHOUTTE, F.; VEREECKE, J.; VERBEKE, N.; et al. Stereoselective effects of the enantiomers of bupivacaine on the electrophysiological properties of the guinea-pig papillary muscle. **British Journal of Pharmacology**; 103: 1275-81, 1991.

ZAPATA-SUDO, G.; TRACHEZ, M.; SUDO, R.T.; NELSON, T. E. - Is Comparative Cardiotoxicity of S(-) and R(+) Bupivacaine Related to Enantiomer-Selective Inhibition of L-Type Ca2+ Channels? **Anesth Analg.** 92(2):496-501, 2001.

APPENDIX - A

Presentations of this work

SATO, R. A comparative study of 0.5% racemic bupivacaine versus 0.5% bupivacaine enantiomeric mixture (S75-R25) in brachial plexus blockade for orthopedic surgery. **American Society of Regional Anesthesia & Pain Medicine, Poster of Annual Fall Pain Meeting & Workshops,** Pointe Hilton, Squaw Peak Resort, Phoenix, AZ. November 11-14, 2004.

SATO, R. T. C.; PORSANI, D. F.; AMARAL, A. G. V.; SCHULZ JR, O. V.; CARSTENS, A. M. G. - Racemic Bupivacaine at 0.5% and Mixture with 50% Enantiomeric Excess (S75-R25) at 0.5% in Brachial Plexus Block for Orthopedic Surgery. Comparative Study. **Brazilian Society of Anesthesiology, Free Theme of the 51st Brazilian Congress of Anesthesiology,** Estaçâo Embratel Convention Center, Curitiba - PR, November 2004.

SATO, R. T. C. - Racemic Bupivacaine at 0.5% and Mixture with 50% Enantiomeric Excess (S75-R25) at 0.5% in Brachial Plexus Block for Orthopedic Surgery. Comparative Study. **Criança 2005, Satellite Symposium of the 2nd International Congress of Pediatric Specialties,** Estaçâo Embratel Convention Center, Curitiba - PR, August 27 to 30, 2005.

SATO, R. T. C. - Racemic Bupivacaine at 0.5% and Mixture with 50% Enantiomeric Excess (S75-R25) at 0.5% in Brachial Plexus Block for Orthopedic Surgery. Comparative Study. **Cristàlia Symposium,** Copas Verdes Hotel, Cascavel - PR, October 27 to 30, 2005.

Publications of this work

SATO, R. A comparative study of 0.5% racemic bupivacaine versus 0.5% bupivacaine enantiomeric mixture (S75-R25) in brachial plexus blockade for orthopedic surgery. **Regional Anesthesia and Pain Medicine**, Vol 30, No 1 (January-February); 108-112, 2005.

SATO, R. T. C.; PORSANI, D. F.; AMARAL, A. G. V.; SCHULZ JR, O. V.; CARSTENS, A. M. G. - Racemic Bupivacaine at 0.5% and Mixture with 50% Enantiomeric Excess (S75-R25) at 0.5% in Brachial Plexus Block for Orthopedic

Surgery. Comparative Study. **Rev Bras Anestesiol**; 55 (2):165 - 174, 2005.

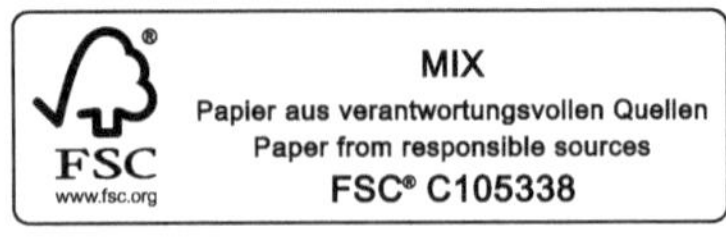

Printed by Books on Demand GmbH, Norderstedt / Germany